HOMEMADE RECIPES THAT KEEP THE HEART HEALTHY

A step by step cooking guide to keep a healthy heart

SOPHIE ANNIE

Table of contents

Breakfast:
1. Oatmeal with Mixed Berries and Almonds
2. Greek Yogurt and Honey Parfait
3. Whole Wheat Pancakes with Fresh Fruit
4. Scrambled Eggs with Spinach and Tomatoes
5. Chia Seed Pudding with Banana Slices
Lunch:
6. Grilled Chicken Salad with Balsamic Vinaigrette
7. Lentil and Vegetable Soup
8. Quinoa and Black Bean Bowl
9. Tuna Salad Wrap with Whole Wheat Tortilla
10. Avocado and Turkey Sandwich
Dinner:
11. Baked Salmon with Lemon and Dill
12. Garlic Shrimp Stir-Fry with Broccoli
13. Grilled Vegetable and Chickpea Quinoa Bowl
14. Skinless Chicken Breast with Roasted Vegetables
15. Baked Cod with Herbed Quinoa
Vegetarian and Vegan Options:
16. Spinach and Mushroom Stuffed Bell Peppers
17. Eggplant Parmesan with Whole Wheat Pasta
18. Vegan Chili with Beans and Veggies
19. Roasted Vegetable and Hummus Wrap
20. Sweet Potato and Black Bean Enchiladas
Snacks:
21. Sliced Cucumber and Hummus
22. Apple Slices with Almond Butter
23. Mixed Nuts and Dried Fruits
24. Greek Yogurt and Blueberries
25. Edamame with Sea Salt

Sides and Salads:
26. Quinoa and Kale Salad with Lemon Dressing
27. Steamed Asparagus with Garlic and Lemon
28. Brown Rice Pilaf with Mixed Herbs
29. Broccoli and Cauliflower Mash
30. Roasted Brussels Sprouts with Balsamic Glaze
Soups:
31. Minestrone Soup with Whole Grain Pasta
32. Tomato Basil Soup with Whole Wheat Croutons
33. Butternut Squash Soup with a Hint of Nutmeg
34. Chicken and Vegetable Rice Soup
35. Gazpacho (Chilled Tomato Soup)
Fish and Seafood:
36. Baked Tilapia with Salsa Fresca
37. Lemon Garlic Shrimp and Zucchini Noodles
38. Tuna Steaks with Mango Salsa
39. Grilled Swordfish with Herb Butter
40. Poached Cod in Tomato Broth
Desserts:
41. Dark Chocolate-Covered Strawberries
42. Mixed Berry Parfait with Low-Fat Yogurt
43. Baked Apples with Cinnamon and Walnuts
44. Banana Ice Cream (Blended Frozen Bananas)
45. Chia Seed and Berry Compote
Smoothies:
46. Spinach and Berry Smoothie
47. Green Tea and Mango Smoothie
48. Tropical Pineapple and Coconut Smoothie
49. Kale and Banana Smoothie
50. Blueberry and Almond Milk Smoothie
—Conclusion

Introduction

In the rhythmic cadence of our lives, amidst bustling schedules and ever-evolving tastes, there exists a universal truth: the profound importance of a healthy heart. It is the tireless sentinel that ensures life's symphony plays on. Your heart beats, on average, over 100,000 times a day, propelling life's vitality through your veins. Thus, it's only fitting that we pay tribute to this wondrous organ by delving into a world of culinary delights specifically designed to nurture and protect it.

Welcome to the culinary odyssey of "Homemade Recipes for a Healthy Heart." In the pages that follow, we will embark on a journey to discover dishes that not only tantalize the taste buds but also fortify the guardian of our vitality – the heart. These recipes are a testament to the fusion of flavor and science, where the ingredients you savor are carefully chosen to promote cardiovascular well-being.

As we navigate through a myriad of sumptuous breakfasts, satisfying lunches, delectable dinners, and guilt-free desserts, you will find that a heart-healthy diet is anything but mundane. It's a celebration of nature's bounty, a harmonious blend of colors and textures that will leave your palate delighted and your heart content.

Breakfast

1. Oatmeal with Mixed Berries and Almonds:

 - **Recipe:**

   - *Ingredients*: Rolled oats, mixed berries (strawberries, blueberries, raspberries), sliced almonds, honey or maple syrup (optional), skim milk or almond milk.

   - *Instructions*: Cook oats with milk according to package directions. Top with sliced almonds, mixed berries, add a drizzle of honey or maple syrup if desired.

   - **How to Eat:** Enjoy this warm, comforting bowl of oatmeal with a spoon. The combination of oats, berries, and almonds provides a satisfying texture and a delightful mix of flavors.

- **Preparation Tips:** Choose unsweetened almond milk or skim milk to keep it low in saturated fat. Opt for fresh or frozen berries, and avoid adding excessive sugar.

2. Greek Yogurt and Honey Parfait:

- **Recipe:**
  - **Ingredients**: Greek yogurt, honey, fresh fruit (e.g., sliced bananas, kiwi, or berries), granola.
  - **Instructions**: Layer Greek yogurt, honey, fruit, and granola in a glass or bowl. Repeat for multiple layers.

- **How to Eat:** Dive your spoon into the layers, ensuring you get a mix of creamy yogurt, sweet honey, fresh fruit, and crunchy granola in each bite.

- **Preparation Tips:** Choose low-fat or non-fat Greek yogurt for a lower saturated fat content. Opt for natural honey without added sugars. Use granola with whole grains and nuts for added fiber.

3. Whole Wheat Pancakes with Fresh Fruit:

- **Recipe:**
  - *Ingredients*: Whole wheat pancake mix, water or skim milk, fresh fruit (e.g., sliced strawberries, blueberries), a drizzle of pure maple syrup.
  - *Instructions*: Prepare whole wheat pancake batter according to package instructions. Cook pancakes on a griddle. Top with fresh fruit and a drizzle of pure maple syrup.

- **How to Eat:** Stack those wholesome pancakes, add fresh fruit on top, and savor the blend of warm, fluffy pancakes with the sweetness of fruit.

- **Preparation Tips:** Opt for whole wheat pancake mix for added fiber. Use a non-stick cooking spray or a small amount of healthy oil to cook the pancakes.

4. Scrambled Eggs with Spinach and Tomatoes:

- **Recipe:**
  - *Ingredients*: Eggs, spinach leaves, diced tomatoes, a pinch of salt and pepper, a touch of olive oil.
  - *Instructions*: In a non-stick skillet, sauté spinach and tomatoes in olive oil. Pour beaten eggs over the veggies. Scramble until cooked through.

- **How to Eat:** Serve the fluffy scrambled eggs with a side of whole grain toast or a slice of whole wheat bread.

- **Preparation Tips:** Use olive oil sparingly for a heart-healthy choice. Consider egg whites if you want to reduce cholesterol intake. Add a dash of hot sauce for extra flavor without adding sodium.

5. Chia Seed Pudding with Banana Slices:

- **Recipe:**
   - **Ingredients**: Chia seeds, almond milk, mashed ripe bananas, a touch of honey (optional), sliced almonds (for garnish).
   - **Instructions**: Mix chia seeds, almond milk, mashed bananas, and honey (if desired) in a jar or container. Stir well and refrigerate

overnight. Top with sliced almonds before serving.

  - **How to Eat:** Scoop out this creamy pudding and enjoy the contrasting textures of chia seeds and banana slices.

  - **Preparation Tips:** Use unsweetened almond milk to keep it lower in sugar. Adjust honey to taste, and consider adding cinnamon for extra flavor.

Lunch:

6. Grilled Chicken Salad with Balsamic Vinaigrette:
  - **Recipe:**
  - *Ingredients*: Grilled chicken breast, mixed greens, cherry tomatoes, cucumber, red onion, bell peppers, balsamic vinaigrette.

- *Instructions*: Toss the ingredients together in a large bowl, drizzle with balsamic vinaigrette, and top with grilled chicken.

- **How to Eat:** Enjoy this vibrant salad with a fork, making sure to get a mix of tender grilled chicken and crisp, fresh vegetables in every bite.

- **Preparation Tips:** Grill chicken without excessive marinades or oils. Opt for a homemade balsamic vinaigrette to control added sugar and sodium.

7. Lentil and Vegetable Soup:

   - **Recipe:**
     - *Ingredients*: Red lentils, carrots, celery, onion, garlic, vegetable broth, a pinch of cumin and paprika.
     - *Instructions*: Sauté vegetables and garlic, add lentils and broth, simmer until tender, and season with cumin and paprika.

   - **How to Eat:** Serve this hearty soup in a bowl, and enjoy it with a side of whole grain bread or a salad.

   - **Preparation Tips:** Use low-sodium vegetable broth to control salt levels. Add a squeeze of lemon for a burst of flavor without extra salt.

8. Quinoa and Black Bean Bowl:

   - **Recipe:**

- *Ingredients*: Cooked quinoa, black beans, corn, diced avocado, cherry tomatoes, cilantro, lime juice.
- *Instructions*: Mix quinoa, black beans, corn, avocado, tomatoes, cilantro, and lime juice in a bowl.

- **How to Eat:** Dig in with a spoon, savoring the fusion of quinoa's nuttiness, black beans' creaminess, and the freshness of lime and avocado.

- **Preparation Tips:** Rinse canned beans to reduce sodium. You can also add a dash of hot sauce for extra flavor without adding salt.

9. Tuna Salad Wrap with Whole Wheat Tortilla:

- **Recipe:**

- *Ingredients*: Canned tuna (in water), Greek yogurt, diced celery, diced red onion, diced pickles, whole wheat tortilla.
- *Instructions*: Mix tuna, Greek yogurt, celery, onion, and pickles. Spread onto a whole wheat tortilla, wrap, and serve.

- **How to Eat:** Fold the tortilla, securing the filling, and enjoy it as a convenient, handheld lunch option.

- **Preparation Tips:** Choose tuna packed in water for a lower-fat option. Greek yogurt adds creaminess without the saturated fat of mayonnaise.

10. Avocado and Turkey Sandwich:

- **Recipe:**

- ***Ingredients***: Sliced turkey breast, avocado, whole grain bread, lettuce, tomato, mustard or a light mayo alternative.
- ***Instructions***: Assemble turkey, avocado, lettuce, and tomato between slices of whole grain bread. Add mustard or a heart-healthy mayo alternative if desired.

- **How to Eat:** Cut the sandwich in halves or quarters and savor each bite with a refreshing crunch.

- **Preparation Tips:** Opt for lean turkey breast without added sodium or preservatives. Whole grain bread should be used for added fiber.

Dinner:

11. Baked Salmon with Lemon and Dill:

- **Recipe:**
   - *Ingredients*: Lemon juice, fresh dill, garlic,salt, olive oil, salmon fillets, and pepper.
   - *Instructions*: Coat salmon with olive oil, lemon juice, garlic, dill, salt, and pepper. Bake until flaky.

- **How to Eat:** Serve the salmon fillet with a side of steamed vegetables and enjoy the delicate flavor with a squeeze of fresh lemon.

- **Preparation Tips:** Baking salmon preserves its heart-healthy omega-3 fatty acids. Fresh dill gives the best flavor.

12.Garlic shrimps stir - fry with broccoli:

- **Recipe:**
  - *Ingredients*: Shrimp, broccoli florets, garlic, ginger, low-sodium soy sauce, sesame oil, red pepper flakes.
  - *Instructions*: Stir-fry shrimp, garlic, and ginger in sesame oil. Add broccoli and soy sauce. Cook until shrimp is pink and broccoli is tender.

- **How to Eat:** Serve this flavorful stir-fry over brown rice or whole wheat noodles.

- **Preparation Tips:** Opt for low-sodium soy sauce to control salt levels. Adjust red pepper flakes to your preferred spice level.

13. Grilled Vegetable and Chickpea Quinoa Bowl:

- **Recipe:**
  - *Ingredients*: Grilled vegetables (zucchini, bell peppers, eggplant), cooked quinoa, chickpeas, lemon-tahini dressing.
  - *Instructions*: Toss grilled vegetables, chickpeas, and quinoa with lemon-tahini dressing.

- **How to Eat:** Enjoy the medley of flavors and textures with a fork in a bowl or as a wrap in a whole wheat tortilla.

- **Preparation Tips:** Grill vegetables with minimal oil. Homemade lemon-tahini dressing lets you control the ingredients and flavor.

14. Skinless Chicken Breast with Roasted Vegetables:

  - **Recipe:**
    - *Ingredients*: Skinless chicken breast, assorted vegetables (e.g., carrots, Brussels sprouts, sweet potatoes), olive oil, herbs.
    - *Instructions*: Season chicken and vegetables with olive oil, herbs, salt, and pepper. Roast or fry until chicken is cooked through or done and vegetables are tender (soft)

  - **How to Eat:** Serve the succulent chicken breast with a generous portion of roasted vegetables for a wholesome meal.

  - **Preparation Tips:** Roasting requires less oil than frying. Season vegetables with your favorite herbs for extra flavor.

15. Baked Cod with Herbed Quinoa:

- **Recipe:**
  - *Ingredients*: Cod fillets, cooked quinoa with herbs, lemon juice, olive oil, garlic, salt, and pepper.
  - *Instructions*: Season cod with olive oil, lemon juice, garlic, salt, and pepper. Bake until flaky. Serve over herbed quinoa.

- **How to Eat:** Delight in the light and flaky cod paired with the fragrant quinoa, using a fork to savor every bite.

- **Preparation Tips:** Baking cod is a heart-healthy choice. Use fresh herbs for a burst of flavor without adding salt.

Vegetarian and Vegan Options:

16. Spinach and Mushroom Stuffed Bell Peppers:

 - **Recipe:**
  - *Ingredients*: Bell peppers, spinach, mushrooms, quinoa, garlic, vegetable broth, and a pinch of red pepper flakes.
  - *Instructions*: Sauté spinach, mushrooms, garlic, and cooked quinoa. Stuff bell peppers with this mixture, bake, and serve.

 - **How to Eat:** Slice into the colorful bell pepper to reveal the delicious stuffing inside, savoring the blend of earthy flavors.

 - **Preparation Tips:** Use vegetable broth with no added sodium for a healthier stuffing base. Adjust red pepper flakes to your spice preference.

17. Eggplant Parmesan with Whole Wheat Pasta:

- **Recipe:**
  - *Ingredients*: Sliced eggplant, whole wheat breadcrumbs, marinara sauce, part-skim mozzarella cheese, whole wheat pasta.
  - *Instructions*: Bread eggplant slices, bake until crisp, layer with sauce and cheese, and bake again until bubbly. Serve over whole wheat pasta.

- **How to Eat:** Cut into the cheesy layers of eggplant Parmesan, enjoying each forkful with whole wheat pasta.

- **Preparation Tips:** Use part-skim mozzarella cheese for a lower-fat option.

Choose whole wheat breadcrumbs and pasta for added fiber.

18. Vegan Chili with Beans and Veggies:

- **Recipe:**
  - *Ingredients*: Kidney beans, black beans, diced tomatoes, onions, bell peppers, chili spices (cumin, paprika, chili powder).
  - *Instructions*: Sauté onions, peppers, and spices. Add beans and diced tomatoes, simmer until flavors meld.

- **How to Eat:** Ladle this vegan chili into a bowl and savor the hearty mix of beans and veggies.

- **Preparation Tips:** Use canned beans with no added salt, and choose diced tomatoes with no added sugar. Adjust spices to taste.

19. Roasted Vegetable and Hummus Wrap:

- **Recipe:**
    - *Ingredients*: Roasted vegetables (zucchini, bell peppers, cherry tomatoes), whole wheat tortilla, hummus.
    - *Instructions*: Fill a whole wheat tortilla with roasted veggies and a generous spread of hummus. Roll and serve.

- **How to Eat:** Bite into the flavorsome wrap, savoring the creamy hummus and the roasted medley of vegetables.

- **Preparation Tips:** Roast vegetables with a drizzle of olive oil. Opt for low-sodium hummus for a healthier wrap.

20. Sweet Potato and Black Bean Enchiladas:

- **Recipe:**
   - *Ingredients*: Sweet potatoes, black beans, whole wheat tortillas, enchilada sauce, cilantro, and lime.
   - *Instructions*: Mash sweet potatoes and black beans, fill tortillas, roll, and place in a baking dish. Top with enchilada sauce, bake, and garnish with cilantro and lime.

- **How to Eat:** Cut into these enchiladas and savor the comforting combination of sweet potatoes and black beans.

- **Preparation Tips:** Use whole wheat tortillas for added fiber. Opt for a lower-sodium enchilada sauce and adjust seasonings to taste.

Snacks:

21. Sliced Cucumber and Hummus:

- **Recipe:**
  - *Ingredients*: Fresh cucumber slices and your choice of hummus.
  - *Instructions*: Simply slice cucumbers and dip them in hummus for a refreshing snack.

- **How to Eat:** Dip cucumber slices in hummus, enjoying the cool crunch of cucumbers paired with the creamy hummus.

- **Preparation Tips:** Opt for plain hummus without added oils or excess salt for a healthier snack.

22. Apple Slices with Almond Butter:

 - **Recipe:**
   - *Ingredients*: Fresh apple slices and almond butter (or other nut butter of your choice).
   - *Instructions*: Slice apples and spread almond butter on each slice.

 - **How to Eat:** Savor the sweet crunch of apples combined with the rich creaminess of almond butter in every bite.

 - **Preparation Tips:** Choose almond butter without added sugars or oils. You can also sprinkle a dash of cinnamon for extra flavor.

23. Mixed Nuts and Dried Fruits:

- **Recipe:**
  - *Ingredients*: A mix of unsalted nuts (almonds, walnuts, cashews) and dried fruits (apricots, raisins, cranberries).
  - *Instructions*: Combine a variety of unsalted nuts with dried fruits in a portable snack bag.

- **How to Eat:** Grab a handful of this energy-boosting mix for a quick and satisfying snack on the go.

- **Preparation Tips:** Choose unsalted nuts to keep sodium intake in check. Be mindful of portion sizes for calorie control.

24. Greek Yogurt and Blueberries:

  - **Recipe:**
    - *Ingredients*: Greek yogurt and fresh blueberries.
    - *Instructions*: Simply top a bowl of Greek yogurt with fresh blueberries.

  - **How to Eat:** Enjoy the creamy, tangy Greek yogurt paired with the burst of sweetness from the blueberries.

  - **Preparation Tips:** Opt for low-fat or non-fat Greek yogurt for a lower saturated fat content. You can also drizzle a touch of honey for extra sweetness.

25. Edamame with Sea Salt:

- **Recipe:**
   - *Ingredients*: Steamed edamame (young soybeans) and a sprinkle of sea salt.
   - *Instructions*: Steam edamame and lightly season with sea salt.

   - **How to Eat:** Pop these nutritious edamame beans from their pods, savoring the natural saltiness.

   - **Preparation Tips:** Steamed edamame is an excellent source of plant-based protein. Use sea salt sparingly for flavor.

Sides and Salads:

26. Quinoa and Kale Salad with Lemon Dressing:

- **Recipe:**
  - *Ingredients*: Cooked quinoa, fresh kale, cherry tomatoes, red onion, lemon dressing (lemon juice, olive oil, garlic).
  - *Instructions*: Toss quinoa, kale, tomatoes, and red onion with the lemon dressing.

- **How to Eat:** Savor the refreshing crunch of kale and the zesty lemon dressing in this satisfying salad.

- **Preparation Tips:** Use a light hand when adding olive oil to the lemon dressing, and adjust garlic to taste.

27. Steamed Asparagus with Garlic and Lemon:

- **Recipe:**
    - *Ingredients*: Fresh asparagus spears, garlic, lemon zest, and lemon juice.
    - *Instructions*: Steam asparagus, then sauté with garlic, lemon zest, and a squeeze of lemon juice.

    - **How to Eat:** Enjoy the tender-crisp asparagus infused with the bright flavors of garlic and lemon.

    - **Preparation Tips:** Steam asparagus with minimal cooking oil. Use lemon zest and juice sparingly to control acidity.

28. Brown Rice Pilaf with Mixed Herbs:

    - **Recipe:**

- *Ingredients*: Brown rice, a mix of fresh herbs, such as parsley, dill, and chives, vegetable broth, and a touch of olive oil.
- *Instructions*: Cook brown rice with vegetable broth, then toss with a variety of finely chopped fresh herbs and a drizzle of olive oil.

- **How to Eat:** Savor each spoonful of this aromatic and herb-infused brown rice pilaf, enjoying the medley of flavors.

- **Preparation Tips:** Choose low-sodium vegetable broth and use olive oil sparingly for a heart-healthy side dish.

29. Broccoli and Cauliflower Mash:

- **Recipe:**

- ***Ingredients***: Steamed broccoli and cauliflower florets, garlic, low-fat Greek yogurt, a pinch of grated Parmesan cheese (optional).

- ***Instructions***: Steam broccoli and cauliflower until tender. Mash with garlic and Greek yogurt. Add a sprinkle of Parmesan cheese if desired.

- **How to Eat:** Spoon into this creamy and nutritious mash, relishing the combination of broccoli and cauliflower.

- **Preparation Tips:** Opt for low-fat Greek yogurt to keep it lower in saturated fat. You can omit the Parmesan cheese for a dairy-free version.

30. Roasted Brussels Sprouts with Balsamic Glaze:

   - **Recipe:**
     - *Ingredients*: Fresh Brussels sprouts, olive oil, balsamic vinegar, a touch of honey (optional).
     - *Instructions*: Toss Brussels sprouts with olive oil, roast until crispy, and drizzle with balsamic glaze (and honey if desired).

   - **How to Eat:** Enjoy these roasted Brussels sprouts with a fork, appreciating the caramelized flavor of the balsamic glaze.

   - **Preparation Tips:** Roast Brussels sprouts with minimal oil. Use honey sparingly for added sweetness.

Soups:

31. Minestrone Soup with Whole Grain Pasta:

- **Recipe:**

- *Ingredients*: Whole grain pasta, kidney beans, diced tomatoes, carrots, celery, onion, garlic, vegetable broth, Italian herbs.

- *Instructions*: Simmer pasta, beans, veggies, and herbs in vegetable broth until cooked.

- **How to Eat:** Savor this hearty minestrone soup with a spoon, enjoying the blend of whole grain pasta and savory vegetables.

- **Preparation Tips:** Use whole grain pasta for added fiber. Opt for low-sodium vegetable broth and canned beans with no added salt.

32. Tomato Basil Soup with Whole Wheat Croutons:

  - **Recipe:**
  - *Ingredients*: Ripe tomatoes, fresh basil, onion, garlic, low-sodium vegetable broth, whole wheat bread (for croutons).
  - *Instructions*: Cook tomatoes, basil, onion, and garlic with vegetable broth. Serve with whole wheat croutons.

  - **How to Eat:** Ladle this comforting tomato basil soup into a bowl and savor the aroma and taste with whole wheat croutons.

  - **Preparation Tips:** Use whole wheat bread for homemade croutons and choose low-sodium vegetable broth.

33. Butternut Squash Soup with a Hint of Nutmeg:

- **Recipe:**
- *Ingredients*: Butternut squash, onion, garlic, vegetable broth, nutmeg, and a touch of Greek yogurt (optional).
- *Instructions*: Cook butternut squash, onion, and garlic with vegetable broth until tender. Blend until smooth. Add a hint of nutmeg and Greek yogurt if desired.

- **How to Eat:** Sip and savor the velvety butternut squash soup with a subtle warmth from the nutmeg.

- **Preparation Tips:** Use a small amount of Greek yogurt for creaminess without adding excess saturated fat.

34. Chicken and Vegetable Rice Soup:

- **Recipe:**
  - *Ingredients*: Skinless chicken breast, carrots, celery, onion, garlic, brown rice, low-sodium chicken broth, thyme.
  - *Instructions*: Simmer chicken, veggies, rice, and thyme in chicken broth. Shred the cooked chicken and serve in the soup.

- **How to Eat:** Enjoy a bowl of this comforting chicken and vegetable rice soup, featuring tender chicken, nutritious veggies, and brown rice.

- **Preparation Tips:** Remove skin from chicken breast for a leaner option. Choose low-sodium chicken broth to control salt levels.

35. Gazpacho (Chilled Tomato Soup):

- **Recipe:**
  - **Ingredients**: Ripe tomatoes, cucumber, bell pepper, red onion, garlic, olive oil, red wine vinegar, fresh basil, and a touch of hot sauce.
  - **Instructions**: Blend all ingredients until smooth. Chill the soup before serving.

- **How to Eat:** Sip this refreshing gazpacho straight from a bowl or a chilled glass, savoring the burst of flavors and the coolness of the soup.

- **Preparation Tips:** Use ripe tomatoes for the best flavor. Adjust hot sauce to your preferred spice level.

Fish and Seafood:

36. Baked Tilapia with Salsa Fresca:

   - **Recipe:**
   - *Ingredients*: Tilapia fillets, salsa fresca (tomatoes, onions, cilantro, lime juice, jalapeño), olive oil.
   - *Instructions*: Season tilapia with olive oil, bake until flaky, and serve with salsa fresca on top.

   - **How to Eat:** Delight in the light and flaky tilapia paired with the zesty and vibrant salsa fresca.

   - **Preparation Tips:** Bake tilapia with minimal oil for a heart-healthy choice. Adjust the jalapeño in the salsa to suit your spice preference.

37. Lemon Garlic Shrimp and Zucchini Noodles:

- **Recipe:**
    - *Ingredients*: Shrimp, zucchini noodles (zoodles), garlic, lemon juice, olive oil, parsley.
    - *Instructions*: Sauté shrimp with garlic and olive oil, toss with zucchini noodles, and drizzle with lemon juice. Garnish with parsley.

- **How to Eat:** Savor the succulent lemon garlic shrimp served over refreshing zucchini noodles, highlighted by the freshness of lemon and parsley.

- **Preparation Tips:** Use olive oil sparingly for a heart-healthy option. Ensure the zucchini noodles are al dente for the perfect texture.

38. Tuna Steaks with Mango Salsa:

  - **Recipe:**
  - *Ingredients*: Tuna steaks, mango salsa (mango, red onion, cilantro, lime juice), olive oil.
  - *Instructions*: Grill or sear tuna steaks with a drizzle of olive oil, and serve with mango salsa.

  - **How to Eat:** Enjoy the mouthwatering tuna steaks, either grilled or seared, paired with the tropical sweetness of mango salsa.

  - **Preparation Tips:** Grill or sear tuna with minimal oil for a heart-healthy choice. Customize the mango salsa ingredients to your taste.

39. Grilled Swordfish with Herb Butter:

- **Recipe:**
   - *Ingredients*: Swordfish steaks, herb butter (butter, fresh herbs, lemon zest), olive oil.
   - *Instructions*: Grill swordfish with a drizzle of olive oil and serve with a dollop of herb butter on top.

- **How to Eat:** Relish the succulent and perfectly grilled swordfish, enhanced by the fragrant herb butter.

- **Preparation Tips:** Grill swordfish with minimal oil. Prepare herb butter with fresh herbs for the best flavor.

40. Poached Cod in Tomato Broth:

- **Recipe:**
  - *Ingredients*: Cod fillets, tomato broth (tomatoes, garlic, onion, vegetable broth), basil, olive oil.
  - *Instructions*: Poach cod in a tomato broth with garlic, onion, and basil. Drizzle with olive oil before serving.

- **How to Eat:** Enjoy tender poached cod immersed in a flavorful tomato broth, accented by the aromatic basil.

- **Preparation Tips:** Use olive oil sparingly for a heart-healthy option. Ensure the cod is cooked to perfection, flaking easily with a fork.

Desserts:

41. Dark Chocolate-Covered Strawberries:

- **Recipe:**
  - *Ingredients*: Fresh strawberries, dark chocolate (70% cocoa or higher).
  - *Instructions*: Melt dark chocolate, dip strawberries, and allow them to cool and harden.

- **How to Eat:** Savor the natural sweetness of strawberries harmonized with the rich depth of dark chocolate in each luscious bite.

- **Preparation Tips:** Choose dark chocolate with a high cocoa content for maximum heart-healthy antioxidants. Use a microwave or a double boiler to melt the chocolate gently.

42. Mixed Berry Parfait with Low-Fat Yogurt:

  - **Recipe:**

  - *Ingredients*: Mixed berries (strawberries, blueberries, raspberries), low-fat yogurt, honey (optional), granola (optional).

  - *Instructions*: Layer low-fat yogurt, mixed berries, honey (if desired), and granola in a glass.

  - **How to Eat:** Delight in the contrasting textures and flavors as you dig into this creamy and fruity parfait.

  - **Preparation Tips:** Opt for low-fat yogurt and use honey sparingly for a healthier option. Choose granola with whole grains and minimal added sugar.

43. Baked Apples with Cinnamon and Walnuts:

- **Recipe:**
   - *Ingredients*: Apples, cinnamon, crushed walnuts, a touch of honey (optional).
   - *Instructions*: Core apples, sprinkle with cinnamon, and top with crushed walnuts. Bake until tender. Drizzle with honey if desired.

- **How to Eat:** Relish the tender warmth of baked apples with a sprinkle of cinnamon and the satisfying crunch of walnuts.

- **Preparation Tips:** Use honey sparingly for added sweetness. Opt for a variety of apples you enjoy.

44. Banana Ice Cream (Blended Frozen Bananas):

   - **Recipe:**
    - *Ingredients*: Ripe bananas.
    - *Instructions*: Slice ripe bananas, freeze until solid, then blend until creamy.

   - **How to Eat:** Enjoy the guilt-free indulgence of banana ice cream, where the natural sweetness of bananas takes center stage.

   - **Preparation Tips:** Freeze bananas when they're perfectly ripe for the best flavor and sweetness.

45. Chia Seed and Berry Compote:

   - **Recipe:**

- ***Ingredients***: Chia seeds, mixed berries (strawberries, blueberries, raspberries), honey, lemon juice.

- ***Instructions***: Mix chia seeds with honey and lemon juice, then let it sit until it thickens. Serve with mixed berries.

- **How to Eat:** Spoon into the chia seed and berry compote, appreciating its delightful blend of textures and natural sweetness.

- **Preparation Tips:** Adjust honey to your preferred sweetness level. Mix the chia seeds well to ensure they absorb the liquid.

Smoothies

46. Spinach and Berry Smoothie:

- **Recipe:**

- *Ingredients*: Fresh spinach, mixed berries (strawberries, blueberries, raspberries), banana, low-fat Greek yogurt, almond milk, honey (optional).
- *Instructions*: Blend spinach, mixed berries, banana, Greek yogurt, almond milk, and honey (if desired) until smooth.

- **How to Enjoy:** Sip on this vibrant green elixir, where the earthiness of spinach blends harmoniously with the sweet and tangy mixed berries.

- **Preparation Tips:** Opt for low-fat Greek yogurt and adjust honey to taste. Add ice cubes for a refreshing chill.

47. Green Tea and Mango Smoothie:

- **Recipe:**
    - *Ingredients*: Green tea (cooled), ripe mango chunks, low-fat Greek yogurt, honey (optional).
    - *Instructions*: Blend cooled green tea, ripe mango, Greek yogurt, and honey (if desired) until smooth.

  - **How to Enjoy:** Relish the soothing and refreshing combination of green tea and the tropical sweetness of mango in each sip.

  - **Preparation Tips:** Brew green tea and allow it to cool before blending. Adjust honey to your preferred sweetness level.

48. Tropical Pineapple and Coconut Smoothie:

- **Recipe:**
    - *Ingredients*: Pineapple chunks, coconut milk, low-fat Greek yogurt, a touch of honey (optional).

- **Instructions**: Blend pineapple, coconut milk, Greek yogurt, and honey (if desired) until smooth.

- **How to Eat** Sip on this tropical paradise in a glass, where the vibrant pineapple meets the creamy coconut.

- **Preparation Tips:** Use unsweetened coconut milk for a healthier option. Adjust honey to your taste preference.

49. Kale and Banana Smoothie:

- **Recipe:**
- **Ingredients**: Fresh kale leaves, ripe banana, almond milk, low-fat Greek yogurt, honey (optional).

- *Instructions*: Blend kale, banana, almond milk, Greek yogurt, and honey (if desired) until smooth.

- **How to Eat:** Savor this nutrient-packed green smoothie, where the earthy notes of kale harmonize with the natural sweetness of banana.

- **Preparation Tips:** Opt for low-fat Greek yogurt and adjust honey to taste. Add a handful of ice cubes for a cooler texture.

50. Blueberry and Almond Milk Smoothie:

- **Recipe:**
- *Ingredients*: Blueberries, almond milk, low-fat Greek yogurt, honey (optional).

- *Instructions*: Blend blueberries, almond milk, Greek yogurt, and honey (if desired) until smooth.

- **How to Enjoy:** Sip on the delightful purple elixir, where the bold flavor of blueberries shines with a touch of creaminess from almond milk and yogurt.

- **Preparation Tips:** Opt for low-fat Greek yogurt and adjust honey to taste. Use unsweetened almond milk for a healthier option.

These recipes offer a delectable array of heart-healthy options that span fish and seafood, indulgent desserts, and revitalizing smoothies. Each dish is an opportunity to relish the blend of flavors and textures while prioritizing your well-being. Adjust these recipes to your dietary preferences and enjoy the journey of culinary creativity intertwined with heart-conscious choices. Bon appétit!

-Conclusion

As our flavorful odyssey through "Homemade Recipes for a Healthy Heart" draws to a close, we stand at the crossroads of culinary delight and cardiovascular wisdom. What we've unearthed is a realm where scrumptious and nutritious unite in a joyful dance on our plates. This journey has been nothing short of a revelation—a symphony of vibrant ingredients, creative recipes, and the very essence of heart-healthy living.

In these pages, breakfasts have awakened our senses, painting our mornings with the comforting strokes of oatmeal adorned with mixed berries and the silky layers of a Greek yogurt and honey parfait. Lunches have invigorated our midday cravings with salads, soups, and wraps that redefine what it means to dine healthily and deliciously. Dinners have been a culinary crescendo, from succulent baked salmon to the zesty waltz of garlic shrimp stir-fry.

For vegetarians and vegans, this journey has been an exploration of culinary innovation, with stuffed bell peppers and hearty vegan chili showcasing that plant-based meals can be as savory and satisfying as any other. Snacks have become more than mere cravings but nutritious pleasures—a crisp cucumber slice dipped in hummus or the sweet crunch of apple slices with almond butter. Our sides and salads have embraced the kaleidoscope of colors and flavors, featuring quinoa and kale salads and balsamic-glazed Brussels sprouts. Even soups have transcended the ordinary, with chilled gazpacho and hearty minestrone taking center stage.

Yet, beyond the culinary adventures, this journey has granted us a profound insight: the connection between our heart's well-being and our choices in the kitchen. A heart-healthy diet isn't a list of "can't haves" but a tapestry of vibrant, life-affirming ingredients. It's about savoring nature's gifts, choosing lean proteins, and respecting portion sizes. It's about appreciating the bounty of fruits and vegetables, experimenting with ancient grains, and cherishing the act of preparing a meal.

As we conclude this chapter, let us remember that our journey towards heart health is an ongoing tale. It's a promise to nourish our hearts not just through food but with acts of self-care, physical activity, and mindfulness. It's a recognition that a heart-healthy lifestyle is a treasure we bestow upon ourselves—a treasure that promises vitality, longevity, and a heart that beats in rhythm with life's most beautiful melodies.

So, let us view these recipes not as an ending but as a prologue to a lifelong culinary voyage—a voyage where the heart is not just fed but celebrated, where every meal is a symphony of love and gratitude for the incredible organ that keeps us alive. Together, we shall savor life's flavors while nurturing the heart that orchestrates our existence. Here's to your heart's health—a symphony of happiness, vibrancy, and the sweet joys of living.